SUN-KISSED TO SUNBURNED

Revealing Sunburn: New Understanding, Effective Methods, and Plans for Taking Control of Your Skin

CHAD BRUNO

Table of Contents

Introductory

Overexposure to ultraviolet (UV) light, either naturally from the sun or artificially via tanning beds, causes sunburn. The DNA in your skin cells can be damaged by UV radiation, which can cause a variety of unpleasant side effects. Redness, discomfort, swelling, and even burning of the skin are all common symptoms of sunburn. The severity of a sunburn ranges from mild to severe depending on factors such as the amount of time spent in the sun and the person's natural pigmentation.

It's crucial to protect your skin from excessive sun exposure to prevent sunburn, as repeated sunburns can increase the risk of skin damage and skin cancer. Sunscreen, hats, long sleeves, and avoiding outside activities during the sun's peak hours are all ways to protect yourself from the sun's harmful rays. If you do get sunburned, you should treat it by applying cold compresses, moisturizing, and taking over-the-counter pain medicines.

The best way to safeguard your skin and overall health when spending time in the sun is to take precautions against being sunburned in the first place.

CHAPTER ONE
The Importance of Wearing Sunscreen

Excessive time in the sun can have negative impacts on your health and well-being, both now and in the future, so it's important to take precautions. Some of the most salient justifications for wearing sun protection are as follows:

• Protection Against Skin Cancer: Melanoma, the worst form of skin cancer, is almost always caused by too much time spent in the sun. Sunscreen is one of the most effective ways to prevent skin cancer.

- Avoiding sunburn is important because getting burned raises your chances of developing skin damage or skin cancer. Sunburns can be avoided with the right precautions, such as the use of sunscreen and the wearing of protective clothes.

- **Early Skin Aging:** Too much time in the sun can hasten the onset of wrinkles, fine lines, age spots, and a general decline in skin elasticity.

- To prevent cataracts and other eye diseases, it's important to shield your eyes from the sun's UV rays. Protecting your eyes by donning UV-blocking sunglasses is crucial.

• Protecting your skin from the sun is important for keeping it healthy and undamaged. Sunspots, actinic keratosis, and the worsening of preexisting skin diseases like rosacea are less likely to occur.

• A sunburn can be quite uncomfortable and even painful. If you take precautions to prevent sun damage to your skin, you can enjoy time spent outdoors without worrying about getting a painful sunburn.

• Some drugs and medical conditions might increase your skin's susceptibility to UV radiation, making it more crucial than ever to use sun protection.

• The UV Index measures the amount of ultraviolet light present at a given place and time of day. You can avoid harmful exposure to the sun by keeping track of the UV index and using suitable sun protection.

• Heat-related disorders, such as heatstroke, can have a negative impact on general health if exposed to the sun for too long. Taking precautions against sun exposure is crucial to maintaining good health.

Here are some things to keep in mind if you want to protect yourself from the sun:

Sunscreen with a high SPF rating and broad-spectrum protection should be used.

Take precautions by donning a hard hat with a brim, a pair of sunglasses, and long sleeves.

• Seek cover during peak solar hours, often between 10 a.m. and 4 p.m.

Water, snow, and sand can all reflect and amplify UV rays, so it's important to take extra precautions around these surfaces.

Avoid heat exhaustion by staying hydrated and taking frequent shade breaks.

Overall, sun protection is a crucial aspect of maintaining good health and preventing the negative effects of UV radiation on your skin and body.

Effects of Skin Type on Susceptibility

Different people have different skin types and therefore be susceptible to different skin problems. Various skin kinds are recognized, each with its unique set of traits and vulnerabilities. The susceptibilities of certain frequently encountered skin types are as follows.

1. Ordinary Skin:

• **Traits:** Normal skin is just the right amount of greasy or dry. The pores are small, the texture is velvety, and the tone is bright.

When compared to other skin types, normal skin is less prone to a wide variety of skin problems. However, it is still vulnerable to the effects of time and environmental variables like ultraviolet radiation.

2. Flaky Skin:

- Dry skin is characterized by a tight, gritty texture and possible flaking or scaling. It may lack natural moisture and may be sensitive.

Dry skin is more prone to wrinkles, fine lines, and skin irritations because of these vulnerabilities. It can also grow more sensitive and prone to disorders like dermatitis.

3. Face Oil:

- Excess sebum production causes oily skin's enlarged pores and glossy appearance. Acne and blackheads are common problems.

Acne, plugged pores, and a shiny appearance are all risks for oily skin. Despite its apparent resistance to the effects of aging, it is not immune to skin problems.

4. Skin Type Combination:

• Traits People with combination skin tend to have an oily T-zone (the area around their nose and chin) and dry or normal cheeks.

Acne in the T-zone and dryness in the cheeks are two examples of the vulnerabilities that might affect people with combination skin.

5. **Traits:** Redness, irritation, and reactions to different skincare products or environmental conditions are all hallmarks of sensitive skin.

• Weaknesses Sensitive skin is easily irritated, which can lead to redness and discomfort. It is sensitive to a wide range of substances and environmental factors.

6. Skin Aging:

• Indications of aging include the appearance of wrinkles, fine lines, a lack of suppleness, and age spots on the skin.

• Weaknesses: Skin's innate fragility makes it more susceptible to the outward manifestations of aging. To preserve its youthful appearance and prevent additional damage, careful care is required.

7. Inflammatory Acne:

• Acne-prone skin is characterized by its propensity to develop pimples, blackheads, and whiteheads.

• Vulnerabilities: Acne-prone skin is subject to persistent acne troubles and eventual scarring. Acne can be controlled with the right skincare routine and medication.

8. A Burn from the Sun:

• Traits Excessive sun exposure causes sun damage, which manifests as uneven pigmentation, age spots, and fine wrinkles.

There is a higher risk of skin cancer, accelerated aging, and more UV damage in skin that has already been affected by the sun.

The key to beautiful, healthy skin is finding the proper products and regimens for your skin type and using them consistently. It's crucial to personalize your skincare technique to your unique skin type and address any particular weaknesses or issues you may have. You can get tailored advice for your skin by consulting with a dermatologist.

CHAPTER TWO
Sunburn: What We Know About It

Overexposure to the sun's ultraviolet (UV) light causes sunburn. Sunburn is the result of a complicated series of physiological and biological reactions in the skin. The most important scientific features of sunburn are as follows:

1. Sunlight emits ultraviolet (UV) radiation; this includes both ultraviolet A (UVA) and ultraviolet B (UVB) photons. Sunburn is typically caused by ultraviolet B (UVB) rays. Exposure to UVB rays causes a cascade of cellular responses in the skin.

2. UVB radiation can cause direct cellular DNA damage to skin cells. Abnormal molecular connections between DNA bases, known as "thymine dimers," are formed. This DNA damage interferes with regular cellular processes and can cause mutations, which may eventually lead to skin cancer.

3. Sunburn causes the skin to go through an inflammatory response. When skin cells are harmed, they release cytokines and other signaling molecules that recruit the body's immune system and widen the blood vessels leading to the injury. Sunburn symptoms including redness and swelling result from this reaction.

4. The production of melanin, the pigment responsible for skin, hair, and eye color, is the skin's natural defense against UV radiation. The skin develops more melanin as a defense mechanism against UV exposure. Although this eventually leads to a tan, it takes time, and too much sun too soon can cause damage to the skin in the form of sunburn.

5. Discomfort and Pain Sunburn results in discomfort and agony as well as peeling skin. This is because a damaged, dry, and overly sensitive skin is the result of the skin's inflammatory response.

6. The entire degree of sunburn may not be evident right away. The worst of the symptoms may not appear for several hours or even a day. Because of this lag, it can be difficult to assess sunburn severity immediately after being exposed to UV rays.

7. Consequences Over time, repeated sunburns and overexposure to UV rays can cause skin damage like wrinkles and age spots, as well as increase the risk of skin cancer and other skin disorders.

8. Protection: Observing sun safety measures is the most effective method for avoiding sunburn. This involves using sunscreen with a high SPF, wearing protective clothes, keeping in the shade during peak sun hours, and avoiding indoor tanning. Sunscreen works by creating a barrier between the skin and the sun, preventing harmful UV rays from penetrating the skin.

Sunburn is a warning indicator of serious skin damage, not simply a little inconvenience. It is essential to take precautions against sunburn and to use sun protection whenever you will be outside in the sun.

The sun and tanning beds are both sources of ultraviolet (UV) radiation, a form of electromagnetic radiation. UV radiation has both beneficial and detrimental effects on living things and the environment. **Key features and consequences of ultraviolet (UV) radiation include the following:**

• In terms of wavelength, ultraviolet light can be roughly classified as follows:

Ultraviolet A (UVA) photons are the least powerful and have the longest wavelength. They cause tanning and can speed up the skin's aging process.

• Medium-wavelength and more powerful than UVA rays are UVB (Ultraviolet B) rays. Sunburns are caused by them, and they also contribute significantly to the growth of skin cancer.

Ultraviolet C (UVC) rays are the most powerful and have the shortest wavelength. The atmosphere of Earth absorbs them, so they never reach the ground.

2. The Upsides:

• Vital to bone health and general well-being, vitamin D is synthesized by the skin in response to UVB exposure.

UVC radiation, which is not present in sunlight, is utilized for sterilizing in a variety of contexts, such as water purification and medical instrumentation.

3. Reversed Benefits:

• Sunburn, accelerated aging, and an upped risk of developing skin cancer are just some of the negative effects of prolonged exposure to ultraviolet (UV) radiation, especially UVA and UVB rays.

• **Eye Damage:** Cataracts and photo keratitis (a painful eye ailment similar to sunburn of the cornea) are two examples of how ultraviolet (UV) radiation can harm the eyes.

• **Immunosuppression:** Exposure to UV radiation can weaken the immune system, leaving people more vulnerable to illness.

Because ultraviolet light may pass through water and injure aquatic life, it poses a threat to aquatic ecosystems. This is especially true of shallow water environments.

4. The harmful effects of ultraviolet (UV) radiation can be reduced by using the following sun protection measures:

• Protect yourself against both UVA and UVB radiation by applying a sunscreen with broad-spectrum protection.

• Wear protective clothing, sunglasses, and wide-brimmed hats to guard the skin and eyes from UV radiation.

• When the sun is at its hottest, at 10 a.m. and 4 p.m.

The intense UV radiation from tanning beds raises the risk of skin cancer, therefore it's best to stay away from them.

5. Protection against ultraviolet (UV) radiation is made possible by the ozone layer above Earth's surface. Ozone layer depletion, caused by human actions like the production of ozone-depleting compounds, has increased the risk of UV exposure at the Earth's surface.

Both good and bad can result from exposure to ultraviolet (UV) radiation; how much damage is done depends on how long someone is in the sun without protection. It is crucial for one's health and well-being to strike a balance between the requirement for UV protection and the benefits of natural UV exposure for vitamin D generation.

CHAPTER THREE
The Signs of Sunburn

In order to treat sunburn and prevent future skin damage, it is crucial to recognize the symptoms. Sunburn symptoms can be mild to severe, and they usually don't show up until several hours after you've been in the sun too long. The following are some of the most obvious symptoms of sunburn:

1. Redness: Sunburned skin appears redder than your regular skin tone. The severity of a sunburn affects how red the skin becomes.

2. Sunburned skin is typically quite delicate and unpleasant to the touch. The pain can start off as a dull ache and progress to a searing inferno.

3. Swelling: If the sunburn is particularly bad, the affected area may swell.

4. Blisters are fluid-filled lumps on the skin that can grow after severe sunburn. These blisters serve as a protective barrier, so please don't pop them.

5. To make matters worse, scratching sunburned skin can

make it much more red and irritated.

6. The afflicted area of skin may begin to peel a few days following the initial sunburn. Your body does this to get rid of dead or damaged skin.

7. Dehydration from too much time in the sun causes sunburned skin to feel dry and tight.

8. Feelings of weariness and discomfort are common among those who have suffered from a severe sunburn.

Keep in mind that sunburn's full severity may not appear right away.

Sunburn's symptoms may not be at their worst until several hours or even a day later. Symptoms may worsen initially before they begin to improve.

Here's what to do if you think you could have sunburn:

1. Avoid further sun exposure by retreating to a cool, shaded spot or going indoors.

2. **Cool the Skin:** Take a cool (not freezing) shower or bath to help calm the skin. Don't use hot water if your skin is in poor shape.

3. Applying a soothing moisturizer, such as aloe vera gel or a mild

lotion, can help alleviate dryness and pain.

4. Because sunburn can cause dehydration, it's important to drink plenty of water after being in the sun.

5. **Pain Relief:** Anti-inflammatory and pain medicines like ibuprofen and acetaminophen are available without a prescription at most drug stores.

6. If you must go outside, protect your skin by wearing protective clothing and sunscreen.

Seek medical treatment if you have blisters, extensive sunburn, or a high temperature from being in the sun. Medical professionals are best equipped to treat and advise on how to manage the issues that can arise from severe sunburn.

Keep in mind that the best way to prevent sunburn is to take preventative measures. Protect your skin from the sun by using sunscreen, wearing protective clothes, and seeking shade during the midday and early afternoon hours.

Shade from the Sun

Sun protection is vital to defend your skin from the harmful effects of ultraviolet (UV) radiation from the sun. Sunburn, accelerated aging, and even skin cancer are all possible outcomes of prolonged exposure to the sun. Key sun safety measures include the following:

1. Put on Sunblock:

A broad-spectrum sunscreen with an SPF of 30 or higher is recommended. Check that it blocks both UVA and UVB radiation.

15-30 minutes before heading outside, liberally apply sunscreen to all areas of exposed skin.

Apply new sunscreen every two hours, or more often if you swim or perspire heavily.

2. Be sure to dress proper safety gear:

o Put on protective clothes, such as long-sleeved shirts, long pants, and hats with wide brims.

Ultraviolet (UV) radiation can damage your skin, so it's important to wear clothing with a UPF rating.

• Sunglasses with UV protection can defend your eyes from UV radiation.

3. Cover up:

Keep out of the sun as much as possible, particularly between 10 a.m. and 2 p.m. and 4 p.m.

Shade yourself from the sun with umbrellas, trees, or anything else you can find.

4. Avoid Indoor Tanning:

A high concentration of UV radiation is emitted by tanning beds, which has been linked to an increased risk of skin cancer. Don't make use of them.

5. Lip balm with sun protection factor (SPF) should be used when going outside in the sun.

6. Avoid dehydration:

In order to avoid becoming dehydrated, you should drink plenty of water before going out in the sun.

7. Watch Out for Mirrors and Windows:

UV rays can be reflected and amplified by water, sand, and snow, increasing your exposure. Be especially careful around these kinds of surfaces.

8. Learn the UV Index:

Keep in mind your area's UV index, which indicates the intensity of UV light. Make the necessary adjustments to your sun protection routine.

9. Sunscreen and Children:

Children are more susceptible to sunburn because of their fair skin. Protect your kids from the sun and the elements by dressing them in layers and applying sunscreen before taking them outside.

10.Skin checks on a regular basis:

- Regularly inspect your skin for any changes, such as new moles, growths, or changes in existing moles. Skin cancer prevention relies on early detection.

11. Continue learning:

- Learn about the risks of overexposure to the sun and how to protect yourself from it.

12. Visit a Skin Doctor:

- Seek professional advice from a dermatologist if you're worried about your skin or have seen any changes.

Keep in mind that UV rays can pass through clouds, so sun protection is necessary even on gloomy or overcast days. By following these sun safety tips, you can spend more time outside without worrying about getting burned or developing skin cancer.

CHAPTER FOUR

How to Choose and Use Sunscreen

Sunscreen is an essential part of sun safety because it protects skin from the sun's damaging ultraviolet (UV) rays. Learn about the different sunscreens and how to apply them correctly for the best results.

Various Sunscreens:

1. Sunscreens that block both UVA and UVB rays are called broad-spectrum. Sunburn is caused by ultraviolet B (UVB) rays, while ultraviolet A (UVA) rays can cause premature skin aging. Sunscreens that block both UVA and UVB rays are called "broad-spectrum."

2. The Sun Protection Factor (SPF) rates how well a sunscreen protects against UVB rays. The higher the sun protection factor (SPF), the better. Common advice calls for an SPF of 30, however longer sun exposure may benefit from a higher SPF.

3. Zinc oxide and titanium dioxide are examples of physical (mineral) sunscreen components. The physical barrier they produce on the skin deflects or scatters the sun's rays. These sunblocks work as soon as they're applied.

4. Sunscreens made of chemical ingredients absorb ultraviolet light and release it as heat. The time it takes for them to start working after being applied is roughly 20-30 minutes. Avobenzone, octisalate, octocrylene, and oxybenzone are just a few of the common chemical sunscreen components.

• Most people don't use nearly as much sunscreen as they should to keep from burning. The recommended amount to cover your complete body is 1 ounce, or the volume of a standard shot glass. A nickel-sized quantity is suggested for use on the face.

• Sunscreen should be applied 15-30 minutes before going outside so that it has time to fully absorb into the skin. This is crucial for chemical sunscreens in particular.

• Don't forget to apply sunscreen on the tops of your feet if they will be uncovered, as well as the ears, neck, and hands.

• Keep Reapplying:

Sunscreen should be reapplied every two hours, or more often if you swim or perspire heavily.

o After drying off completely, even if the sunscreen is "water-resistant."

Please remember to reapply after you've had anything to eat or drink..

• Use lip balm with SPF to protect your lips.

Use sunscreen religiously, but pay special attention to your nose and cheeks, which burn easily.

• Protect yourself against both UVA and UVB radiation by applying a broad-spectrum sunscreen.

• Sunscreen that has passed its expiration date may not provide the same level of protection. Use new sunscreen every time.

• Protecting yourself from the sun involves more than just using sunscreen. The best way to protect yourself from the sun is to stay indoors, wear dark clothing, and avoid going outside between the hours of 10 a.m. and 4 p.m.

• **Pick the Right SPF Value:** Sunscreens with higher SPF values offer additional protection, but no product can guarantee complete safety. When spending a lot of time outside, it's best to use an SPF of 30 or greater.

• Applying sunscreen is something you should do consistently, not just in the summer. Even on overcast days, UV rays can penetrate.

In order to prevent sunburn, skin damage, and skin cancer, sunscreen must be applied correctly. Remember that sunscreen should be one element of a comprehensive sun protection approach that includes protective clothing and seeking shade when necessary.

A Remedy for Sunburn

Relieving discomfort, minimizing skin damage, and speeding healing are all reasons to treat sunburn. Here are some tips to help you deal with and heal from sunburn:

1. First, you should get out of the sun and into some shade or an air-conditioned room right away. Avoiding more solar damage is dependent on this step.

2. Take a cool (not cold) shower or bath to soothe your skin. When applied to sunburned skin, this can help calm the area and reduce pain. Stay away from hot water, since it may make your situation more worse.

3. For 15-20 minutes at a time, apply cool, moist washcloths or compresses to the burnt regions. The heat and ache can be alleviated with this.

4. Moisturize the skin by rubbing in some aloe vera gel or a mild moisturizer (one without alcohol). This may alleviate symptoms by decreasing dryness.

5. Drinking water helps prevent sunburn, which can cause dehydration.

6. Nonsteroidal anti-inflammatory medicines (NSAIDs) such as ibuprofen or aspirin are available without a prescription and can be used to treat pain, inflammation, and discomfort. Always refer to the label for proper dosage.

7. Stay away from Anything That Could Cause Further Irritation To Your Sunburned Skin. Avoid using anything that contains alcohol, perfume, or any other irritants.

8. If blisters appear as a result of sunburn, it is essential that you do not pop them. Blisters create a protective barrier that can help avoid infection.

9. Keep the burnt areas covered to prevent further skin damage from the sun. Clothes that are loose but tightly woven should be worn to hide the damaged regions.

10. **Avoid Sunbathing:** Do not attempt to "even out" your tan by obtaining more sun exposure. This can make the burn much more severe and lead to more skin damage.

11. To avoid illness, avoid getting your skin sunburned. Be on the lookout for signs of infection, such as spreading redness, pus, or intensifying discomfort, and be sure to keep the afflicted areas clean.

12. To alleviate irritation and scratching, your doctor may suggest a topical corticosteroid cream. These are for usage under a physician's supervision only.

13. Sunburns that are particularly painful, affect a wide area of the body, or are accompanied by other symptoms such as a high temperature, chills, or persistent pain should be evaluated by a medical expert.

Keep in mind that it may take several days for sunburn to recover entirely, so it's important to take precautions and minimize sun exposure during this time. Sunburn is a sign of skin damage, and repeated sunburns can increase the chance of skin cancer, therefore it's crucial to practice sun safety to prevent future occurrences.

CHAPTER FIVE
First-Aid Measures and Home Remedy

Sunburn causes pain and agony, but there are home remedies and first aid procedures that can help alleviate such symptoms. Sunburn can be extremely painful, but these home treatments will help ease the pain and speed up the healing process. Here are some tried-and-true first aid techniques and home cures for sunburn:

1. Apply cool, wet compresses or washcloths to the burnt regions. The heat and soreness can be relieved with this. Don't use ice because it's very abrasive for your skin.

2. A cool (not chilly) shower or bath might help relieve pain and discomfort. Instead of touching your skin, pat it dry with a fresh towel.

3. Use aloe vera gel on your sunburned skin. The anti-inflammatory and healing characteristics of aloe vera make it useful for easing skin irritation.

4. Sunburn can cause dehydration, therefore it's important to drink enough of water to prevent that.

5. Over-the-Counter Pain Relief: Non-prescription pain medications like ibuprofen or aspirin can help reduce pain and inflammation. Always refer to the label for proper dosage.

6. Apply a mild, alcohol-free moisturizer to the skin to keep it supple and hydrated. Creams containing hydrocortisone may also help relieve inflammation and irritation.

7. A chilly bath containing colloidal oatmeal can be quite relaxing for the skin. Oatmeal-based soaps and shampoos are sold at pharmacies.

8. Paste made from baking soda and water can be applied on sunburns for relief. The itching and pain may subside after doing this.

9. Slices of cucumber, or mashed cucumber, can be applied to sunburned skin for a cooling and soothing effect.

10. Sunburn relief: some people find that putting raw potato slices on their skin helps.

11. Sunburned skin can benefit from the anti-inflammatory and healing properties of witch hazel.

12. Brew some green tea, let it cool, and then use the compress to soothe your sunburn. Green tea's antioxidants are great for the skin.

13. Vinegar Soak: Take a cool bath with a cup of white vinegar added to it. It has the potential to ease the pain of sunburn.

14. Wearing loose-fitting garments can protect burnt skin from chafing and increased aggravation.

15. Avoid more sun exposure if your skin has already been burnt. Make sure to cover up and find someplace cool to rest.

Keep in mind that while these cures may help, they are no substitute for avoiding sunburn in the first place.

Sun safety measures, such as applying sunscreen, wearing protective clothes, and seeking shade when appropriate, are essential for preventing sunburn in the first place. Seek medical help for examination and treatment if your sunburn is severe, covers a significant region, or causes serious symptoms.

Sunburn's Long-Term Consequences

Sunburn, especially repeated sunburns over the course of a lifetime, can have lasting effects on the skin and the body. The risk of sunburn can be reduced by being aware of these potential outcomes and practicing sun protection. Sunburn can have lasting consequences such as:

1. Skin injury: Sunburn signifies acute skin injury resulting from excessive exposure to UV radiation. Repeated sunburns can cause chronic skin damage, making the skin more prone to signs of aging such as wrinkles, fine lines, and a lack of elasticity.

2. Sunburn increases your risk of developing skin cancer, which is a serious and life-threatening condition. Damage to skin cells' DNA caused by sun exposure, especially from UVB rays, is a known risk factor for the development of skin cancer. Individuals with a history of sunburns have an increased risk of developing skin cancer, particularly melanoma (the most lethal form of skin cancer).

3. Skin Discoloration: Sunburns can lead to the development of brown patches, often known as age spots or sunspots, on the skin. These tend to become more obvious as people get older.

4. Actinic keratosis is a precancerous skin condition characterized by rough, scaly patches on the skin, and sunburns can lead to its development. Actinic keratosis has the potential to develop into cancer if left untreated.

5. Reduced Resistance to Infection, Itching, and Other Skin Problems UV radiation can reduce the body's capacity to repair and protect the skin, leaving it vulnerable to infections, irritations, and other skin problems.

6. Damage to the Eyes Prolonged exposure to the sun can cause cataracts and photokeratitis, which cause discomfort in the cornea and feels like a sunburn.

7. Enhanced Sensitivity: Sunburn increases the skin's sensitivity, which can contribute to the development of other skin disorders like eczema or rosacea.

8. Aesthetic Decline: Sunburned skin can age unevenly, increasing the likelihood of dryness, roughness, and pigmentation problems.

9. Damage to the skin, darkening of the skin, and the onset of skin diseases are all apparent repercussions of sunburn that can have a negative effect on a person's sense of self-worth and general happiness.

10. People who have already suffered sunburn may be more susceptible to further burns since their skin is now more delicate and fragile.

Sun safety should be a top priority to reduce the risk of long-term skin damage from sun exposure. Sunscreen with a high SPF, protective clothes, and seeking cover during the middle of the day are all great ways to avoid sun damage to your skin. You can lessen your chances of being sunburned and suffering from its aftereffects by adopting these habits and limiting your time spent outdoors.

CHAPTER SIX
Factors to Take Into Account

Different criteria, such as age, skin type, and medical issues, necessitate different approaches to sunburn and sun protection.

1. Particular care must be taken to prevent sunburn in children because their skin is more delicate. Sunscreen and protective gear designed for children should be used, and they should be kept in the shade during the hottest parts of the day. Keep infants younger than six months away of the sun.

2. Elderly People: Skin becomes more prone to sun damage and cancer as we age. Older people should take extra care to protect themselves from the sun. Checking your skin often might help you see changes early on.

3. In terms of sunburn and skin damage, persons with pale skin are at a disadvantage versus those with darker complexion, whose higher melanin content acts as a natural sunscreen. Even those with darker skin tones need to take precautions to avoid sunburn.

4. Sensitivity to the sun may be exacerbated by medical conditions or drugs. Antibiotics, acne treatments, and medical diseases like lupus are just a few examples of how skin might become more sensitive to the sun. In these situations, it's best to seek the advice of a medical professional.

5. During pregnancy, a woman's skin may become more or less sensitive to the sun. Hormonal shifts make the skin more prone to pigmentation changes, including the "mask of pregnancy" (melasma), therefore it's necessary to take safeguards.

6. People who have a family history of skin cancer, especially melanoma, should take extreme precautions to avoid sun exposure. It is crucial to visit a dermatologist regularly for skin exams and follow-up.

7. Some people may be allergic to the components in sunscreen, or they may have sensitivities to the sun. In such circumstances, hypoallergenic sunscreens are available. Allergies can be diagnosed with the use of a patch test.

8. Prolonged sun exposure may occur in certain vocations. Outdoor workers, such as construction workers and farmers, should take extra care, including wearing protective gear, using sunscreen, and seeking shade during breaks.

9. Sunburn danger increases with both altitude and latitude: closer to the equator and at higher elevations. Sun protection is especially important at high altitudes and close to the equator.

10. After a recent sunburn, your skin may still be more sensitive even though it may look healed. Keep using sunscreen, as your skin's new layer may be more susceptible to the sun.

11. Everyone's skin is different, and some people may be more or less sensitive to the sun than others. Consider how your skin reacts to sun exposure before deciding how to protect it.

The most important thing is to take precautions and avoid overexposure to the sun, taking into account your specific environment and skin type. If you have questions or concerns regarding sunburn, sunscreen, or your skin in general, talk to your doctor or a dermatologist.

Sun Protection Measures and Precautions

Protecting your skin from sunburn, avoiding skin damage, and decreasing your risk of getting skin cancer all begin with a commitment to prevention and sun safety routines. Key sun safety procedures include the following:

1. Put on Sunblock:

Broad-spectrum sunscreen with an SPF of 30 or higher is recommended.

15-30 minutes before heading outside, liberally apply sunscreen to all areas of exposed skin.

Sunscreen should be reapplied every two hours, or more often if you swim or perspire heavily.

2. Be sure to dress proper safety gear:

• Put on protective clothes, such as long-sleeved shirts, long pants, and hats with wide brims.

Ultraviolet (UV) radiation can damage your skin, so it's important to wear clothing with a UPF rating.

• Wear sunglasses with UV protection to shield your eyes from UV rays.

3. Cover up:

Keep out of the sun as much as possible, particularly between 10 a.m. and 2 p.m. and 4 p.m.

Shade yourself from the sun with umbrellas, trees, or anything else you can find.

4. Avoid Indoor Tanning:

A high concentration of UV radiation is emitted by tanning beds, which has been linked to an increased risk of skin cancer. Don't make use of them.

5. Lip balm with sun protection factor (SPF) should be used when going outside in the sun.

6. Avoid dehydration:

In order to avoid becoming dehydrated, you should drink plenty of water before going out in the sun.

7. Watch Out for Mirrors and Windows:

UV rays can be reflected and amplified by water, sand, and snow, increasing your exposure. Be especially careful around these kinds of surfaces.

8. Learn the UV Index:

• Keep in mind your area's UV index, which indicates the intensity of UV light. Make the necessary adjustments to your sun protection routine.

9. Sunscreen and Children:

Children are more susceptible to sunburn because of their fair skin. Protect your kids from the sun and the elements by dressing them in layers and applying sunscreen before taking them outside.

10. Skin Checks On A Regular Basis: Regularly inspect your skin for any changes, such as new moles, growths, or changes in existing moles. Skin cancer prevention relies on early detection.

11. Continue learning:

• Learn about the risks of overexposure to the sun and how to protect yourself from it.

12. Visit a Skin Doctor:

• Seek professional advice from a dermatologist if you're worried about your skin or have seen any changes.

Keep in mind that UV rays can pass through clouds, so sun protection is necessary even on gloomy or overcast days. Taking these precautions will allow you to comfortably enjoy the outdoors without worrying about becoming sunburned, damaging your skin, or even developing skin cancer.

CHAPTER SEVEN

Skin Maintenance in General

Taking care of your skin on a regular basis is crucial if you want your complexion to glow. Taking care of your skin includes incorporating various aspects of your daily routine and way of life. The following are essential steps in any skin care routine:

1. Remove dirt, makeup, and other impurities from your skin by cleansing it twice a day (morning and night). Choose a mild cleanser that is pH-balanced and ideal for your skin type.

2. In order to remove dead skin cells and encourage new skin growth, exfoliating the skin a couple of times a week is recommended. The texture of your skin and the effectiveness of subsequent treatments can both benefit from exfoliation.

3. Keeping your skin hydrated and protected from dryness can be as simple as using a good moisturizer. It's important to find a moisturizer that works well with your skin.

4. Protection from the sun: Apply sunscreen with an SPF of at least 30 every day, even on overcast ones. The sun's ultraviolet (UV) rays are a leading cause of skin aging, wrinkles, and cancer.

5. The skin around your eyes is very thin, so it's important to take special care of it with an eye cream. Try to find one that works on the specific signs of aging you wish to address.

6. Fine lines, hyperpigmentation, and acne are just some of the skin issues that can be addressed with the help of serums. Select serums that contain active ingredients that help with your concerns.

7. Diet and Hydration: Maintain a balanced diet rich in vitamins and antioxidants. Drink plenty of water to keep your skin hydrated from the inside out.

8. Get a good night's rest. Lack of sleep can cause problems with the skin, such as dark circles under the eyes and a lackluster appearance.

9. Products with harsh or irritating ingredients should be avoided, and any allergens or triggers for your skin should be avoided as well.

10. If you care about your skin's health and appearance, you should steer clear of cigarettes and booze.

11. Meditation and yoga are great stress relievers that can help you avoid the skin problems that can arise from stress.

12. Makeup brushes and sponges can harbor bacteria and cause skin irritation if not cleaned regularly.

13. Take a shower after working out to get rid of sweat and prevent your pores from getting clogged.

14. Do not exfoliate too often; doing so can irritate the skin. Exfoliate gently and at the suggested intervals.

15. When in doubt about your skin type or if you have persistent skin problems, it's best to get a professional opinion from a dermatologist.

It's important to remember that different skin types and concerns require different approaches to skin care. One person's "perfect" solution might not be right for another. It could take some time to find the right routine and products for you, so please be patient. Maintaining healthy and beautiful skin requires a consistent effort to care for the skin.

Expert Skin Care

When it comes to your skin's health and appearance, it's best to leave it in the hands of trained professionals like dermatologists, estheticians, and other specialists who have years of experience in the field. These experts provide comprehensive care for your skin by treating a wide variety of issues. Some components of expert skin care include:

1. Dermatologists are medical doctors who focus on skin care, specifically skin cancer, acne, eczema, psoriasis, and other skin conditions. In extreme cases, they can even perform surgery or prescribe medications on a medical level.

2. Estheticians are skin care experts who use specialized training and products to help clients look and feel their best. They offer a variety of services, including facials, chemical peels, microdermabrasion, and extractions. Estheticians advise clients on how to best care for their skin at home and recommend products.

3. Treatments from experts Skin care experts provide a variety of treatments tailored to individual needs. Laser therapy, chemical peels, microdermabrasion, dermaplaning, and microneedling are just some of the possible

procedures that fall under this category. Fine lines, wrinkles, hyperpigmentation, and acne scars are just some of the cosmetic concerns that can be addressed with these treatments.

4. Professionals can customize a skin care regimen for your specific skin type and address your specific skin care concerns. They will know what services and goods will work best for you.

5. Professionals often have access to high-end skincare equipment and technology that is out of reach for most consumers. Effective treatments for a wide range of skin

issues are within reach with the help of this apparatus.

6. Important for the early detection and prevention of skin cancer, dermatologists can perform screenings for the disease.

7. Acne and rosacea, for example, often require stronger medications, such as retinoids or antibiotics, that can only be obtained with a doctor's prescription.

8. Learning About Your Skin Type and the Best Products and Treatments for It is Possible with the Help of a Professional Skin Care Advisor.

9. Visits to your dermatologist or esthetician at regular intervals will allow you to track your skin's progress and make any necessary adjustments to your care plan.

10. Dermatologists are trained to identify and treat a wide range of skin conditions, such as eczema, psoriasis, and dermatitis.

When looking for professional skin care services, it's critical to find people who can be trusted. Look for proof of legitimacy, such as certifications and licenses, as well as testimonials from satisfied customers. Communication with your skincare professional is also crucial, so you can discuss your goals and concerns and work together to develop an effective and safe skin care plan.

Conclusion

Sunburn is a common but entirely preventable skin condition caused by excessive exposure to ultraviolet (UV) radiation from the sun. Redness, pain, and an increased risk of skin cancer are just a few of the unpleasant short-term effects that may occur. Sunburn and UV damage can be prevented by taking sun safety precautions like applying sunscreen, donning protective clothing, seeking shade, and avoiding tanning beds.

General skin care practices like cleansing, moisturizing, and exfoliating, in addition to sun protection, can aid in keeping skin healthy and radiant. It is important to take immediate first aid measures when dealing with sunburn, such as cooling the skin, applying moisturizers, and staying hydrated. Sun safety and moderate sun exposure are crucial because sunburn can cause permanent skin damage and raise the risk of skin cancer.

Sun protection measures should be adjusted for those with special needs, such as children, those with fair or dark skin, and those with certain medical conditions. Dermatologists and estheticians offer professional skin care services to help improve skin health and target specific issues.

The skin is the body's largest organ, so keeping it healthy is essential to living a long and happy life. Maintaining and protecting your skin can help you achieve and maintain healthy, beautiful skin for years to come. This can be done through daily sun safety habits, general skin care routines, or professional assistance.

THE END